NATIONAL HEALTH INEQUALITY MONITORING
A STEP-BY-STEP MANUAL

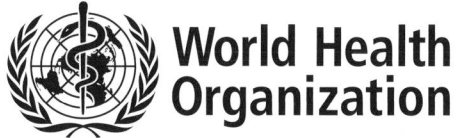

National health inequality monitoring: a step-by-step manual

ISBN 978-92-4-151218-3

© **World Health Organization 2017**

Some rights reserved. This work is available under the Creative Commons Attribution-NonCommercial-ShareAlike 3.0 IGO licence (CC BY-NC-SA 3.0 IGO; https://creativecommons.org/licenses/by-nc-sa/3.0/igo).

Under the terms of this licence, you may copy, redistribute and adapt the work for non-commercial purposes, provided the work is appropriately cited, as indicated below. In any use of this work, there should be no suggestion that WHO endorses any specific organization, products or services. The use of the WHO logo is not permitted. If you adapt the work, then you must license your work under the same or equivalent Creative Commons licence. If you create a translation of this work, you should add the following disclaimer along with the suggested citation: "This translation was not created by the World Health Organization (WHO). WHO is not responsible for the content or accuracy of this translation. The original English edition shall be the binding and authentic edition".

Any mediation relating to disputes arising under the licence shall be conducted in accordance with the mediation rules of the World Intellectual Property Organization.

Suggested citation. National health inequality monitoring: a step-by-step manual. Geneva: World Health Organization; 2017. Licence: CC BY-NC-SA 3.0 IGO.

Cataloguing-in-Publication (CIP) data. CIP data are available at http://apps.who.int/iris.

Sales, rights and licensing. To purchase WHO publications, see http://apps.who.int/bookorders. To submit requests for commercial use and queries on rights and licensing, see http://www.who.int/about/licensing.

Third-party materials. If you wish to reuse material from this work that is attributed to a third party, such as tables, figures or images, it is your responsibility to determine whether permission is needed for that reuse and to obtain permission from the copyright holder. The risk of claims resulting from infringement of any third-party-owned component in the work rests solely with the user.

General disclaimers. The designations employed and the presentation of the material in this publication do not imply the expression of any opinion whatsoever on the part of WHO concerning the legal status of any country, territory, city or area or of its authorities, or concerning the delimitation of its frontiers or boundaries. Dotted and dashed lines on maps represent approximate border lines for which there may not yet be full agreement.

The mention of specific companies or of certain manufacturers' products does not imply that they are endorsed or recommended by WHO in preference to others of a similar nature that are not mentioned. Errors and omissions excepted, the names of proprietary products are distinguished by initial capital letters.

All reasonable precautions have been taken by WHO to verify the information contained in this publication. However, the published material is being distributed without warranty of any kind, either expressed or implied. The responsibility for the interpretation and use of the material lies with the reader. In no event shall WHO be liable for damages arising from its use.

Design and layout by L'IV Com Sàrl, Villars-sous-Yens, Switzerland.
Printed in Luxembourg.

Contents

Foreword iv

Acknowledgements v

How to use this resource 1

Health inequality monitoring: a brief overview 3

STEP ❶ Determine scope of monitoring 7
    Overview 9
    A. Decide on health topics 10
    B. Identify relevant health indicators 11
    C. Identify relevant dimensions of inequality 12
    Examples and resources 14

STEP ❷ Obtain data 17
    Overview 19
    A. Conduct data source mapping 20
    B. Determine whether sufficient data are currently available 21
    Examples and resources 22

STEP ❸ Analyse data 25
    Overview 27
    A. Prepare disaggregated data 28
    B. Calculate summary measures of inequality 29
    Examples and resources 30

STEP ❹ Report results 33
    Overview 35
    A. Define the target audience and purpose of reporting 36
    B. Select the scope of reporting 37
    C. Define the technical content of the report 38
    D. Decide upon methods of presenting data 39
    E. Adhere to best practices of reporting 40
    Examples and resources 41

Glossary 42

Flow chart 45

Foreword

In many ways, the Millennium Development Goals were successful in reducing poverty-related development gaps between countries. The United Nations 2030 Agenda for Sustainable Development (2016–2030) takes this further, promoting greater equity between and within countries, benefiting populations and individuals everywhere. The Sustainable Development Goals (SDGs) contain strong unambiguous language about the importance of equity. The SDG on health is no exception. Universal health coverage is considered the key target to make significant progress towards the SDG on health and well-being for all at all ages. Universal health coverage is about reaching all communities and people with high-quality services, including promotion, prevention, treatment and care, without incurring financial catastrophe. No one can take for granted progress towards the equity dimension of universal health coverage and the broader SDG agenda. The importance of health inequality monitoring within countries, and globally, is paramount.

Monitoring health and health interventions in disadvantaged populations is challenging for many countries. One difficult challenge lies in improving policies and programmes based on monitoring and evaluation of health policies, programmes and practices that target disadvantaged population subgroups. Successfully applying the results of monitoring and evaluation for sustained improvement is necessary to reach the ambitious SDG targets.

Health inequality monitoring should be a central component of national health information systems. Surprisingly, however, national health information systems often neglect to capture within-country inequalities. Sometimes this can be addressed by more effectively communicating existing analyses and underlying disaggregated data to the appropriate target audiences. At other times, it requires expanded or more rigorous analysis of existing data. And sometimes, improving the quality, scope and reach of data collection efforts is needed. Countries should be strategic in planning how to most effectively collect relevant data through routine systems, surveys or special studies to understand the health inequalities within the population.

This manual serves as a step-by-step practical reference to support countries in building capacity for integrating health inequality monitoring into their health information systems. It presents a range of World Health Organization tools and resources developed for measuring and reporting health inequality. As such, this manual aims to contribute to improved monitoring of health inequalities in countries, a practice that is essential to ensure accountability for the goals and targets of the United Nations 2030 Agenda for Sustainable Development.

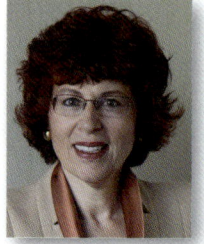

Flavia Bustreo
Assistant Director-General
Family, Women's and Children's Health Cluster
World Health Organization

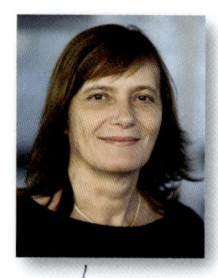

Marie-Paule Kieny
Assistant Director-General
Health Systems and Innovation Cluster
World Health Organization

Acknowledgements

Ahmad Reza Hosseinpoor (World Health Organization, Geneva, Switzerland) and Nicole Bergen (Faculty of Health Sciences, University of Ottawa, Ottawa, Canada) conceptualized and developed the manual.

Early drafts of the manual benefited from the contributions of the following reviewers:

- Aluisio JD Barros, Cesar Victora (International Center for Equity in Health, Federal University of Pelotas, Pelotas, Brazil)
- Nunik Kusumawardani (National Institute of Health Research and Development, Ministry of Health, Jakarta, Indonesia), Mahlil Ruby (Centre for Health Economic and Policy Studies, University of Indonesia, Depok, Indonesia), Sabarinah (Faculty of Public Health, University of Indonesia, Depok, Indonesia)
- Theadora Swift Koller, Veronica Magar, Frank Pega, Anne Schlotheuber, Nicole Valentine (World Health Organization, Geneva, Switzerland)
- Oscar Mujica (Pan-American Health Organization/World Health Organization Regional Office for the Americas, Washington DC, United States)
- Christine Brown, Tina Dannemann Purnat, Claudia Stein (World Health Organization Regional Office for Europe, Copenhagen, Denmark)
- Hala Abou-Taleb, Arash Rashidian, Zafar Ullah Mirza (World Health Organization Regional Office for the Eastern Mediterranean, Cairo, Egypt)

AvisAnne Julien provided copy-editing support and proofread the document.

Funding for the project was provided in part by the World Health Organization, the Regional Office for South-East Asia and the Country Office for Indonesia.

This work is the product of a collaboration between the Information, Evidence and Research Department and the Gender, Equity and Human Rights Team at the World Health Organization.

Sustainable Development Goals and the importance of health inequality monitoring

The United Nations 2030 Agenda for Sustainable Development aspires to *leave no one behind*. This commitment is reflected throughout the 17 Sustainable Development Goals (SDGs), which are integrated and indivisible. The reduction of inequalities is articulated explicitly in SDG 10 (to reduce inequality within and among countries) and is also evident in SDG 1 (to end poverty), SDG 4 (to ensure inclusive and equitable quality education), SDG 5 (to achieve gender equality) and others. SDG 3 is a call to ensure healthy lives and promote well-being for all at all ages, which implies tackling inequalities in health.

Strong national health inequality monitoring systems are fundamental for countries to be accountable that no one is being left behind on the road to sustainable development. Health inequality monitoring is a practice that is part of the national health information system. It serves to identify population subgroups that are disadvantaged, and to track progress on how health improvements (or changes) are realized. For instance, health inequality monitoring has a role in the achievement of universal health coverage (SDG target 3.8), which aims to provide people with the health care they need without suffering financial hardship. The progressive realization of universal health coverage is tracked through health inequality monitoring: optimally, accelerated gains are realized in disadvantaged populations, thus narrowing coverage gaps as the health of the broader population improves.

The 2030 Agenda for Sustainable Development recognizes the importance of strong data and information systems. SDG 17, focusing on strengthening the means of implementing sustainable development initiatives, underscores the importance of increasing the availability of disaggregated data that are high quality, timely and reliable (SDG target 17.18).

How to use this resource

The *National health inequality monitoring: a step-by-step manual* was designed to serve as a highly accessible, practical reference for the practice of health inequality monitoring. Organized according to a flow chart, the manual helps readers to anticipate and navigate practical considerations that underlie health inequality monitoring.

The overarching goals of the *National health inequality monitoring: a step-by-step manual* are: to assist with the establishment of health inequality monitoring systems in countries where it is not currently conducted; to strengthen this practice in countries where it is conducted; and to encourage all countries to integrate regular health inequality monitoring into their national health information systems. Through this resource, we aim to strengthen capacity for health inequality monitoring across settings with varied priorities, capabilities, resources and/or data availability. Further, we hope that this manual will foster regular reporting of inequalities in diverse health topics, and encourage greater integration of the results of health inequality monitoring within policies, programmes and practices.

While the manual focuses on health at the national level, the approach may be applied to monitor inequalities within any defined population, ranging from a community context to a multinational context.

Following a brief introduction to health inequality monitoring, the manual is organized around four main sections, each devoted to one step of health inequality monitoring. The steps form the basis of a flow chart for the practice of health inequality monitoring. In each of the four sections, an expanded version of the flow chart (which is included in full at the end of the manual) displays sub-steps, key questions and itemized checklists of data requirements, analysis/reporting activities and/or decision points. The fifth step, which covers implementing changes based on the results of health inequality monitoring, is addressed in the following section "Health inequality monitoring: a brief overview".

Guidance is provided through brief, practically oriented texts and, where applicable, sample templates. In addition, the manual outlines pertinent examples and resources at each step, with recommended references for more in-depth exploration of issues related to health inequality monitoring. A glossary provides a quick reference for key terminology encountered throughout the manual.

The manual was designed to be read sequentially and in its entirety, however, some readers may find it useful to consult sections of the manual as required. Readers are encouraged to supplement the manual with other reading and educational materials that provide more details on the theoretical aspects of health inequality monitoring. In particular, the *Handbook on health inequality monitoring: with a special focus on low- and middle-income countries* is recommended as the primary resource to complement the content of this manual. Geared towards a broad audience interested in expanding their general knowledge about the practice of health inequality monitoring, the *Handbook* follows the same steps as this manual, offering a more comprehensive discussion about the theory that underlies each step and incorporating practical examples. Throughout the manual, references to specific sections of the *Handbook* will direct readers to relevant material in this companion resource. Note that the *Handbook* has also been adapted into an eLearning format to facilitate a dynamic learning experience.

For online versions of these resources, see:
- Handbook on health inequality monitoring: with a special focus on low- and middle-income countries at: www.who.int/gho/health_equity/handbook/en/; in Spanish at: http://iris.paho.org/xmlui/handle/123456789/31211
- Health inequality eLearning module at: extranet.who.int/elearn/course/category.php?id_15

Health inequality monitoring: a brief overview

Health inequality monitoring can be explained by breaking the term down into its two constituents: health inequality; and monitoring. **Health inequalities** are defined as observable health differences between subgroups within a population, and **monitoring** is a process of repeatedly observing a situation to watch for changes over time. Health inequality monitoring identifies where inequalities exist and where disadvantaged subgroups (demographically, economically, geographically or socially) stand in terms of health. When health inequalities are determined to be unjust, unfair and avoidable, they are referred to as **health inequities**.

Monitoring health inequality requires two types of data: data about health; and data about **dimensions of inequality**. The concept of health is construed broadly for the purpose of monitoring. Depending on the desired scope of monitoring, it may encompass one or more specific health topics and/or capture other diverse aspects of the health sector (including the health workforce, health financing, health information and service delivery, as well as proximate determinants such as water and sanitation, air pollution, etc.). For a given health topic, **population subgroups** may have different experiences according to age, economic status, education level, place of residence, race or ethnicity, sex, social status or other characteristics. These characteristics, known as dimensions of inequality or **equity stratifiers**, reflect social, economic, geographical, demographic or other characteristics that may serve as a basis for discrimination within a population.

When conducted regularly, health inequality monitoring can help to determine the impact of policies, programmes and practices, and to inform necessary changes to reduce inequality. Health inequality monitoring is an important component of health situation analyses, and can also help countries and territories track action on the social determinants of health. Thus, health inequality monitoring serves an essential public health function, and should be institutionalized as a regular practice of national health information systems.

Health inequality monitoring can be conceptualized as a 5-step cycle:

1. The process begins by selecting relevant health topics (which may also capture broader aspects of the health sector), and then identifying a broad range of health indicators and dimensions of inequality that are pertinent to those health topics and the population under consideration.

2. The second step involves obtaining data about those health indicators and inequality dimensions from one or more data sources.

3. Data are then analysed to generate information, evidence and knowledge. The process of analysing health data can include calculating health estimates by population subgroups (that is, **disaggregated estimates**) and **summary measures of inequality**.

④ Following analysis, it is essential to report and disseminate the results. The goal of this step is to ensure that the results of the monitoring process are communicated effectively, and can be used to inform policies, programmes and practices.

⑤ Based on monitoring results, changes may be implemented that will impact and improve health. In order to monitor the effects of these changes, more data must be collected that describe the ongoing state of health; thus, the cycle of monitoring is continual.

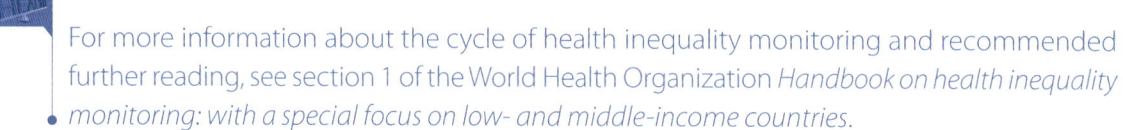

For more information about the cycle of health inequality monitoring and recommended further reading, see section 1 of the World Health Organization *Handbook on health inequality monitoring: with a special focus on low- and middle-income countries*.

Figure 1. Health inequality monitoring flow chart

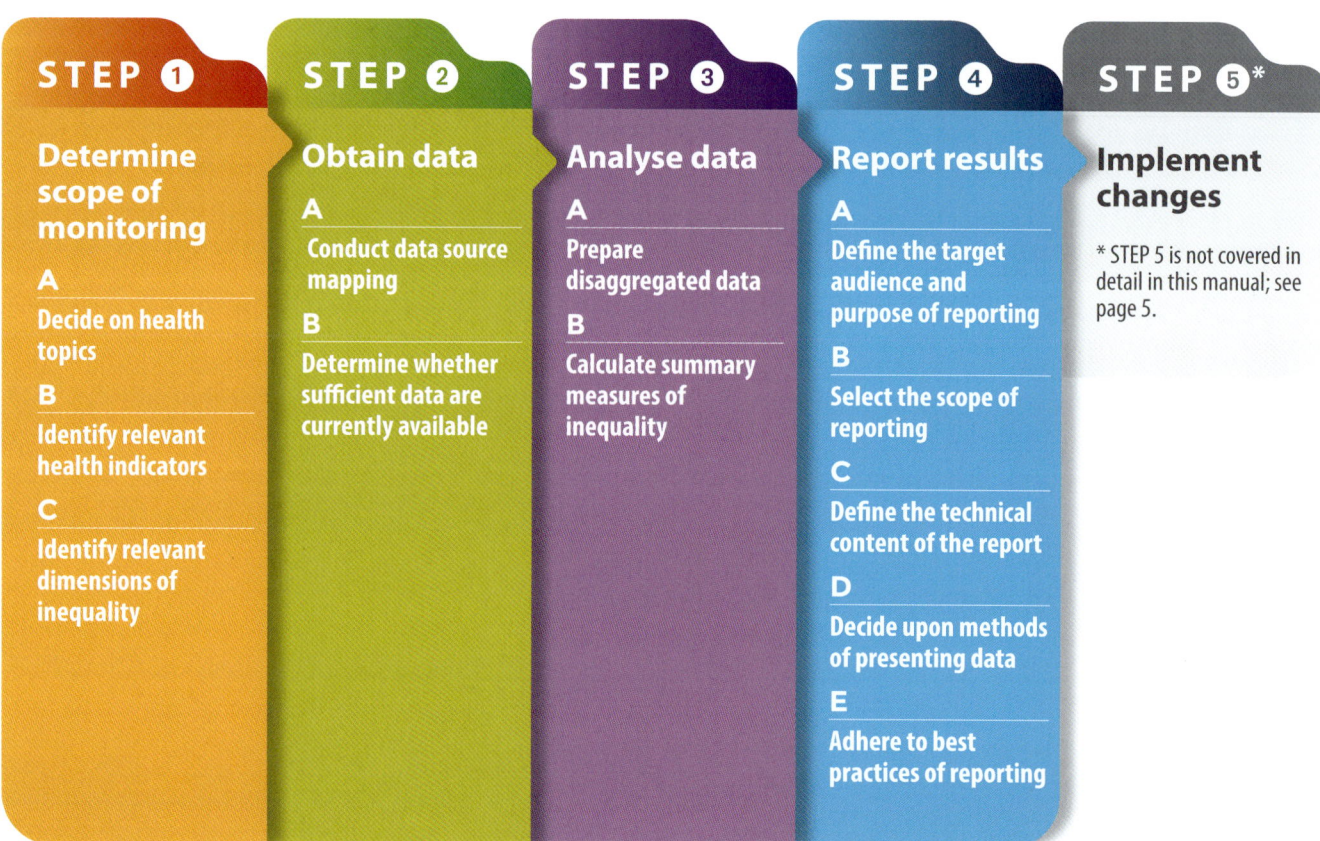

This manual primarily focuses on the first four steps of the cycle, which are each broken down into a series of sub-steps (Figure 1). The progression through steps 1–4 is a complex undertaking that requires consideration of important conceptual issues; the general nature of this progression, however, can be presented in the logical and linear design of a flow chart. The fifth step of the health inequality monitoring cycle, which focuses on implementing change, is highly context specific and iterative. It requires multiple types of inputs to effect change in policies, programmes and practices. An in-depth exploration of this fifth step is not within the scope of this manual. Fortunately, a number of other resources address the complexity of setting priorities based on the results of health inequality monitoring, and applying results within policy and programmatic settings.

> **See**
>
> "Implementing changes based on the results of health inequality monitoring" below

Implementing changes based on the results of health inequality monitoring

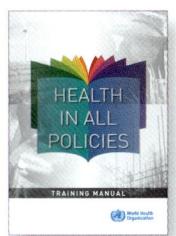

The results of health inequality monitoring is one of several inputs that can help policy-makers to determine priority areas for further action, and/or inform national health policy agendas. Stakeholders with expertise in health data and statistics should review health inequality reports and, incorporating other sources of quantitative and qualitative data, make evidence-based recommendations. Given that health inequalities are frequently shaped by factors beyond the health system, addressing health inequalities may require intersectoral action, such as a Health in All Policies approach.

- For more information about Health in All Policies, see: apps.who.int/iris/bitstream/10665/151788/1/9789241507981_eng.pdf

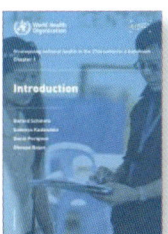

Implementing changes to address health inequalities requires action across levels of the health system and at cross-governmental levels. A strategic entry point is through national health policies, strategies and plans, which should promote the reduction of health inequalities, especially through programme planning and implementation as well as budgetary allocations. Further, the results of health inequality monitoring should be incorporated into situation assessments, priority setting/prioritization processes, and monitoring, evaluation and review approaches. Targets linked to strategic directions and key objectives for the health sector should be equity oriented.

- For more information about national health policies, strategies and plans, see: *Strategizing national health in the 21st century: a handbook* at: http://www.who.int/healthsystems/publications/nhpsp-handbook/en/

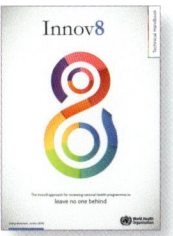

The *Innov8 approach for reviewing national health programmes to leave no one behind: technical handbook*, developed by the World Health Organization, guides the application of health inequality monitoring results to national health programming. The Innov8 approach is an 8-step, sequential review methodology that helps countries to systematically and comprehensively orient the delivery and design of health programmes to ensure that they leave no one behind. Drawing from the results of health inequality monitoring, this approach guides multidisciplinary review teams through an extensive process yielding a better understanding of the causes of health inequities. It helps to identify entry points in programmes to make them more equity oriented, rights based and gender responsive as well as to address critical social determinants. Further, the methodology encourages stakeholders to integrate measures to achieve sustained change and improved governance and accountability. The Innov8 approach can be adapted and applied in diverse settings and to different levels of governance.

- For the *Innov8 approach for reviewing national health programmes to leave no one behind: technical handbook* and other supporting materials, see: http://www.who.int/life-course/partners/innov8/en

STEP 1

Determine scope of monitoring

STEP 1	STEP 2	STEP 3	STEP 4	STEP 5
Determine scope of monitoring	Obtain data	Analyse data	Report results	Implement changes

STEP 1
Determine scope of monitoring

A
Decide on health topics

KEY QUESTION
What are current priority health topics?

CHECKLIST
- What are the objectives identified in health sector planning regarding priority health topics, and/or other broader aspects of the health sector that require assessment?
- How are resources being invested to improve health?
- Which health topics are currently not being monitored, but should be?

B
Identify relevant health indicators

KEY QUESTION
What package of health indicators aptly reflects the health topics?

CHECKLIST
- Select a package of indicators that includes both health interventions and health outcomes
- Identify indicators that cover components of the Monitoring, Evaluation and Review Framework:
  - inputs and processes
  - outputs
  - outcomes
  - impact
- Consider including tracer (or proxy) indicators, and if feasible, composite indicators

C
Identify relevant dimensions of inequality

KEY QUESTION
What dimensions of inequality are relevant in this population, given the selected health topics?

CHECKLIST
- Consider common factors that facilitate disadvantage:
  - economic status
  - education level
  - place of residence
  - sex
  - age
  - other country or context-specific factors
- Consider whether dimensions of inequality intersect, and if double disaggregation should be done
- For each inequality dimension identified above, determine the criteria for how to measure it

Overview

STEP ❶ of health inequality monitoring begins by selecting one or more relevant health topics (which may capture focused health topics and/or broader aspects of the health sector), and then identifying health indicators and dimensions of inequality that are pertinent to those topics and the population under consideration. This step may be political, as it entails consultation with diverse stakeholders that are involved with matters related to health and health determinants. Stakeholders may include technical staff from ministries of health and statistical offices, policy-makers, researchers, health-care professionals, civil society groups, nongovernmental organizations, funding institutions and others. To inform this step, take stock of existing reports and literature – health sector progress and performance reports, and annual health statistical reports, if available, can be used as a basis – as well as advocacy efforts that pertain to health inequalities. These sources may provide evidence that supports the selection of health topics, health indicators and dimensions of inequality.

 For more information about the first step of health inequality monitoring, see section 1 of the World Health Organization *Handbook on health inequality monitoring: with a special focus on low- and middle-income countries*.

A. Decide on health topics

STEP 1

Determine scope of monitoring

A Decide on health topics

B Identify relevant health indicators

C Identify relevant dimensions of inequality

KEY QUESTION
What are current priority health topics?

CHECKLIST
- What are the objectives identified in health sector planning regarding priority health topics, and/or other broader aspects of the health sector that require assessment?
- How are resources being invested to improve health?
- Which health topics are currently not being monitored, but should be?

The selection of health topics (or topic) for inequality monitoring will depend on the desired scope. For instance, establishing a comprehensive national health inequality monitoring system entails an expansive scope, covering numerous health topics (vertical focus), all aspects of the health sector (horizontal focus) and their intersection. For other purposes, it may be appropriate to focus on a narrower selection of health topics, or even a single topic. Some common health topics that constitute a vertical focus include: reproductive, maternal, newborn, child and adolescent health; noncommunicable diseases; injuries; tuberculosis; HIV/AIDS; malaria; and neglected diseases. Examples of a horizontal focus include: health status; service delivery; health workforce; health information; health financing and health governance; as well as proximate determinants such as water and sanitation, air pollution, etc.

> **See**
> "Examples of packages of health indicators" on page 14

The objectives of health sector planning and how resources are being invested (for example, by the health sector and/or government) may signal where there is already political support for establishing or strengthening health inequality monitoring practices. Depending on the purpose of health inequality monitoring, it may be appropriate to select a topic that is already highly visible, or one that has been unduly neglected. For less visible topics, data availability may be an issue.

B. Identify relevant health indicators

STEP 1

Determine scope of monitoring

A Decide on health topics

B Identify relevant health indicators

C Identify relevant dimensions of inequality

KEY QUESTION

What package of health indicators aptly reflects the health topics?

CHECKLIST

☐ **Select a package of indicators that includes both health interventions and health outcomes**

☐ **Identify indicators that cover components of the Monitoring, Evaluation and Review Framework:**
  - inputs and processes
  - outputs
  - outcomes
  - impact

☐ **Consider including tracer (or proxy) indicators, and if feasible, composite indicators**

To get a full sense of the health topic(s) (which may capture specific health topics and/or broader aspects of the health sector), it is important that the health indicator package include diverse types of health indicators related to both health interventions and health outcomes. This core set of health indicators should reflect the needs and interests of the country, but may draw from established indicators that have a common international definition.

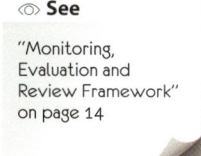

See "Monitoring, Evaluation and Review Framework" on page 14

The **Monitoring, Evaluation and Review Framework** developed by the World Health Organization organizes health indicators into four components: inputs and processes; outputs; outcomes; and impact. Within each component, various categories of indicators are defined that allow the measurement of health at many levels. For monitoring of expansive health topics (such as national health sector monitoring), select indicators from all four components; for a narrower selection of health topics, certain input and process indicators may be less relevant.

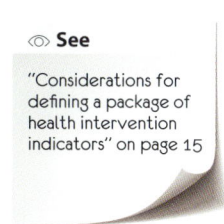

See "Considerations for defining a package of health intervention indicators" on page 15

Using tracer, proxy or composite indicators are concise ways to track progress or performance in a health topic. **Tracer indicators** are highly specified health indicators, chosen to represent a broader health topic. Where data availability is limited or a desired indicator is currently difficult to measure, the use of **proxy indicators** may be a viable consideration. Proxy indicators can provide useful insight, but should be considered an interim solution. A **composite indicator** is an index composed of several indicators within a health topic thereby providing a more comprehensive overview than a single indicator.

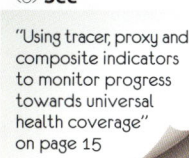

See "Using tracer, proxy and composite indicators to monitor progress towards universal health coverage" on page 15

C. Identify relevant dimensions of inequality

STEP 1

Determine scope of monitoring

A Decide on health topics

B Identify relevant health indicators

C **Identify relevant dimensions of inequality**

KEY QUESTION

What dimensions of inequality are relevant in this population, given the selected health topics?

CHECKLIST

☐ **Consider common factors that facilitate disadvantage:**
  ○ economic status
  ○ education level
  ○ place of residence
  ○ sex
  ○ age
  ○ other country or context-specific factors

☐ **Consider whether dimensions of inequality intersect, and if double disaggregation should be done**

☐ **For each inequality dimension identified above, determine the criteria for how to measure it**

See "Monitoring, Evaluation and Review Framework: considerations for selecting relevant dimensions of inequality" on page 16

To identify **dimensions of inequality**, consider which are relevant to the population and health topic(s) at hand; that is, what types of factors constitute a source of discrimination or social exclusion that may be detrimental to health. Dimensions of inequality that are frequently applied in health inequality monitoring (and recommended by the 2030 Sustainable Development Agenda as bases for data disaggregation) include: income; gender; age; race; ethnicity; migratory status; disability; and geographic location (urban/rural). In addition, education is a common global dimension of inequality. Other factors that may be relevant in a given country or context include subnational region, religion, occupation and indigenous status.

In some cases, two or more dimensions of inequality may intersect and result in exacerbated disadvantage or may reveal a different pattern of inequality than indicated by either single dimension of inequality. **Double disaggregation** entails considering two dimensions of inequality simultaneously when forming subgroups for monitoring. For example, the urban poor typically experience much higher levels of disadvantage than the urban rich. For health inequality monitoring, it may be relevant to identify rich and poor subgroups within urban populations. The comparisons of these two subgroups may be much more striking than comparisons based on either dimension considered separately. Other combinations of dimensions of inequality, such as sex and economic status, may also indicate relevant intersections. For example, in some settings the socioeconomic gradient of smoking is opposite in men and women. In these cases (and others), double disaggregation is warranted for a more meaningful exploration of health inequalities.

At this stage, also consider what criteria will be used to measure each dimension of inequality. These criteria will be specific to the dimension of inequality and type of information that is available about the population. For instance, in low- and middle-income countries, economic status is commonly measured as household wealth whereas in high-income countries economic status can be defined by individual income level.

> **See**
>
> "Defining population subgroups based on economic status" on page 16

Examples and resources

Examples of packages of health indicators

In 2015, the World Health Organization published a standard set of 100 core health indicators, serving as a general reference and guide for standard indicator definitions. The set of indicators takes into account global health priorities specified in the United Nations Millennium Development Goals agenda, as well as emerging priorities laid out in the post-2015 Sustainable Development Goals. This global set of indicators may serve as a useful starting point when determining pertinent health topics for monitoring, though this list was not intended to limit the extent of monitoring. Countries should also consider other health priorities. The *Global reference list of 100 core health indicators* covers the following topics:

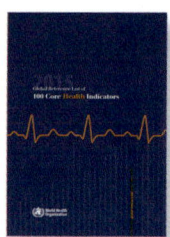

Health status: mortality by age and sex; mortality by cause; fertility; morbidity

Risk factors: nutrition; infections; environmental risk factors; noncommunicable diseases; injuries

Service coverage: reproductive, maternal, newborn, child and adolescent; immunization; HIV; HIV/TB; tuberculosis; malaria; neglected tropical diseases; screening and preventive care; mental health

Health systems: quality and safety of care; access; health workforce; health information; health financing; health security

- For the *Global reference list of 100 core health indicators*, see: http://apps.who.int/iris/bitstream/10665/173589/1/WHO_HIS_HSI_2015.3_eng.pdf?ua=1

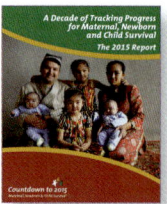

Other sets of health indicators have been proposed for monitoring of specific health topics. For instance, the Countdown to 2015 initiative (now Countdown to 2030) conducts regular monitoring of a set of key indicators related to maternal, newborn and child survival. Equity analyses and profiles reflect the results of health inequality monitoring across Countdown countries.

- For the Countdown reports, see: http://countdown2030.org/

The Global Strategy for Women's, Children's and Adolescents' Health (2016–2030) has developed an indicator and monitoring framework to advance women's, children's and adolescents' health, in line with the United Nations 2030 Agenda for Sustainable Development. The framework identifies 60 indicators to track progress towards the global strategy, as well as a minimum subset of 16 key indicators within three focal areas: survive; thrive; and transform.

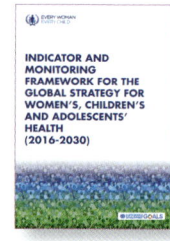

- For the *Indicator and monitoring framework for the Global Strategy for Women's, Children's and Adolescents' Health (2016–2030)*, see: http://www.who.int/life-course/about/coia/indicator-and-monitoring-framework/en/

Monitoring, Evaluation and Review Framework

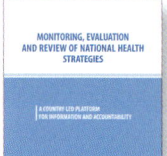

The Monitoring, Evaluation and Review Framework, developed by the World Health Organization in 2011, provides guidance for strengthening monitoring, evaluation and review of national health plans and strategies.

- For the *Monitoring, evaluation and review of national health strategies: a country-led platform for information and accountability*, see: http://www.who.int/healthinfo/country_monitoring_evaluation/1085_IER_131011_web.pdf

For more information about the application of the Monitoring, Evaluation and Review Framework to health inequality monitoring, including an illustration of how the topic of reproductive, maternal, newborn and child health is represented across the four components of the Framework, see section 1 of the World Health Organization *Handbook on health inequality monitoring: with a special focus on low- and middle-income countries*.

Considerations for defining a package of health intervention indicators

Epidemiological relevance: The indicator should reflect an intervention that is associated with a significant burden of disease or potential burden of disease. For indicators of preventive interventions (such as immunization coverage), the relevance may be determined based on the mortality or morbidity prevented by the intervention.

Cost-effective intervention: There should be an evidence base showing that the intervention is effective and feasible to deliver.

Measurable numerator: The numerator reflects the population that received the intervention. Records from health facilities and/or respondents in health surveys should be able to accurately report about the provision or receipt of the intervention. The intervention should be well defined so that records and recall are unambiguous.

Measurable denominator: The denominator reflects the population that needed the intervention. The denominator is easiest to measure when the whole population requires the intervention; for treatment coverage, the denominator – the number of people with the condition – may be more difficult to determine.

Target: The intervention indicator should have an ultimate target of 100% coverage. That is, the goal should be that the denominator (the number of people who need the intervention) should equal the numerator (the number of people who receive the intervention).

Ability to disaggregate: The health indicator should be able to be disaggregated by common dimensions of inequality such as sex, economic status, education, area of residence, etc.

Quality: The health indicator should reflect an intervention that is delivered with a level of quality to achieve the desired outcome.

Comparable: The indicator should be measured in a manner that is comparable over time and across countries.

Easy to communicate: Indicators must be easy to communicate to the intended audience.

Data availability: Indicators should have high-quality, comparable data. Data are often derived from sources such as population-based surveys or health facility records.

Inclusion in international initiatives: When possible, include indicators that are recommended and used in international initiatives, such as United Nations General Assembly or World Health Assembly resolutions.

Source: Adapted from: Boerma T, AbouZahr C, Evans D, Evans T. Monitoring intervention coverage in the context of universal health coverage. PLoS Med. 2014;11(9):e1001728. doi:10.1371/journal.pmed.1001728.

Using tracer, proxy and composite indicators to monitor progress towards universal health coverage

Developed by the World Health Organization and the World Bank, a framework to monitor progress towards universal health coverage (part of the Sustainable Development Goal on health) demonstrates the application of tracer, proxy and composite indicators. The framework covers the two major components of universal health coverage: coverage of quality essential health services; and coverage of financial protection from out-of-pocket health expenses. The proposed indicator to capture coverage of quality essential health services is a composite indicator: an index of national service coverage. The coverage index combines data about a set of 16 tracer indicators. The tracer indicators capture essential health services within four categories: reproductive, maternal, newborn and child health; infectious diseases; noncommunicable diseases; and service capacity and access, and health security. The national service coverage index is calculated as the average across the 16 tracer indicators (first calculating the average in each of the four categories, and then calculating the average of the four category scores). Certain indicators serve as proxy measures. For instance, the prevalence of non-raised blood pressure and mean fasting plasma glucose are used as proxies for hypertension and diabetes treatment, respectively, until analyses are completed to allow for direct reporting on treatment coverage.

- For more information about monitoring progress towards universal health coverage, see:
  - Boerma T, AbouZahr C, Evans D, Evans T. Monitoring intervention coverage in the context of universal health coverage. PLoS Med. 2014;11:e1001728.
  - Hogan D, Hosseinpoor AR, Boerma T. Developing an index for the coverage of essential health services. Technical note. Geneva: World Health Organization; 2016 (http://www.who.int/healthinfo/universal_health_coverage/en/).

Monitoring, Evaluation and Review Framework: considerations for selecting relevant dimensions of inequality

Certain considerations arise when determining which dimensions of inequality are relevant across the four components of the Monitoring, Evaluation and Review Framework. For example, inputs and processes indicators are sometimes defined at the national level (such as health financing, governance and information); if defined at the subnational level, then they can be disaggregated by relevant inequality dimensions (for example, health workforce can be disaggregated by geography). Outputs indicators are normally disaggregated by geography along with other setting-specific relevant dimensions. Outcomes indicators can be disaggregated by four or five common inequality dimensions, plus any relevant setting-specific ones. Impact indicators can be disaggregated by four or five common inequality dimensions, plus any relevant setting-specific ones.

 Defining population subgroups based on economic status

Economic status, a dimension of inequality that is commonly applied when doing health inequality monitoring, can be constructed using various approaches. Challenges arise when attempting to construct a globally applicable common measure for economic status, as the constructs of economic status differ between high-income countries and low- and middle-income countries. Individual (or household) income is among the preferred metrics of economic positioning in high-income countries (where remuneration is more likely to be in monetary form, and received through formal employment), whereas household asset indices – reflecting ownership of durable goods and household characteristics – may be a more feasible measurement in low- and middle-income countries. Consumption data relate to the final use of goods and services, and are primarily obtained through collecting expenditure data. This is the primary methodology used for international poverty monitoring.

- For more information about the metrics used to define population subgroups by economic status, see:
  - O'Donnell OA, Wagstaff A. Analyzing health equity using household survey data: a guide to techniques and their implementation. Washington DC: World Bank Publications; 2008.
  - Howe LD, Galobardes B, Matijasevich A, Gordon D, Johnston D, Onwujekwe O et al. Measuring socio-economic position for epidemiological studies in low- and middle-income countries: a methods of measurement in epidemiology paper. Int J Epidemiol. 2012;41(3):871–6.

STEP 2

Obtain data

STEP 2
Obtain data

A
Conduct data source mapping

KEY QUESTION
What sources contain data about the health indicators and dimensions of inequality?

CHECKLIST
- ☐ List available data sources by type (including name, year, etc.)
- ☐ For each data source, determine availability of data for dimensions of inequality
- ☐ For each data source, determine availability of data about health indicators
- ☐ Combine the information about health indicators and dimensions of inequality to assess data availability for health inequality monitoring

B
Determine whether sufficient data are currently available

KEY QUESTION
Are appropriate data available about both health indicators and dimensions of inequality to proceed with health inequality monitoring?

CHECKLIST
- ☐ Assess the findings from the data source mapping exercise in STEP 2A
- ☐ Consider whether data from different sources may be linked

Overview

STEP ❷ of health inequality monitoring is to source data about the health indicators and dimensions of inequality. To complete this step you will need information about the data sources that exist in your jurisdiction. It is important to understand the strengths and limitations of the available sources to ensure that the best available data are used for health inequality monitoring. Ideally, data should come from an information-producing system that: has strong legitimacy; has high-level political support; is transparent; and includes policy, technical, academic and civil society constituencies. Data representativeness should be taken into account: nationally representative data may be used for national monitoring, whereas data representative of a specific region or a small survey may be used for subnational monitoring.

The practice of health inequality monitoring is an iterative process. This second step of health inequality monitoring may require a return to the first step if, for example, data sources are inadequate or data are of low quality for the indicators selected in STEP 1. Alternative indicators or proxy indicators may need to be considered. Similarly, indicators may not be able to be adequately disaggregated by the selected dimensions of inequality. Encountering these types of barriers provides insight into how health information systems may need to be strengthened, and where additional data collection is warranted.

The approach to obtaining data described below enables users to create a series of lists, cumulating in a final table that demonstrates sources that contain data about both health indicators and dimensions of inequality. Then, users determine whether sufficient data are currently available for health inequality monitoring.

For more information about the second step of health inequality monitoring, see section 2 of the World Health Organization *Handbook on health inequality monitoring: with a special focus on low- and middle-income countries.*

A. Conduct data source mapping

STEP 2

Obtain data

A Conduct data source mapping

B Determine whether sufficient data are currently available

KEY QUESTION

What sources contain data about the health indicators and dimensions of inequality?

CHECKLIST

☐ List available data sources by type (including name, year, etc.)

☐ For each data source, determine availability of data for dimensions of inequality

☐ For each data source, determine availability of data about health indicators

☐ Combine the information about health indicators and dimensions of inequality to assess data availability for health inequality monitoring

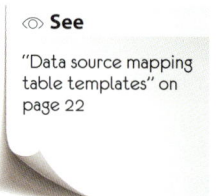

◉ See
"Data source mapping table templates" on page 22

◉ See
"Major data sources and their strengths and limitations" on page 24

The process of **data source mapping** outlined below involves preparing a series of four connected tables, which demonstrate the availability of data across different data sources. Data source mapping begins by creating a list showing available data by source type (census, administrative/facility, household survey, vital registration, etc.), data source name, and year(s) of data collection. A column may be added for notes, such as the frequency of data collection, or the data representativeness. This list forms the first table.

The next stage involves creating an expanded second table showing the availability of data about dimensions of inequality within these data sources. The focus here is on the relevant dimensions of inequality identified in STEP 1C. For easy reference in the next parts of the process, number each row. Use check marks to indicate when data are contained within the data source. In creating this table, it is important to recognize that different data may be available in different years for a given data source.

The third table lists priority health indicators that pertain to the health topic (as identified in STEP 1B), and indicates whether they are described within the various data sources. Use the data source row number (as indicated in the previous list) to show the data sources that contain data on each indicator.

Finally, create a fourth table using the information from the previous two lists. The list of health indicators (in rows), as directly above, should be the starting point. From here, construct columns for each of the relevant dimensions of inequality. In the cross cells, indicate the data source numbers that are common to each health indicator and dimension of inequality combination.

B. Determine whether sufficient data are currently available

STEP 2

Obtain data

A Conduct data source mapping

B **Determine whether sufficient data are currently available**

KEY QUESTION

Are appropriate data available about both health indicators and dimensions of inequality to proceed with health inequality monitoring?

CHECKLIST

☐ **Assess the findings from the data source mapping exercise in STEP 2A**

☐ **Consider whether data from different sources may be linked**

The results of the data source mapping exercise in STEP 2A identify data sources that contain the two types of data for health inequality monitoring. In such cases, provided that sufficient data are available and of high quality, health inequality monitoring can proceed. It is also possible that data about health and data about dimensions of inequality may come from different data sources that can be **linked.** Data linking is done through identifiers (linkages) that exist in both data sources, allowing health indicator and dimension of inequality data to be merged. Data may be linked at the level of the individual (for example, based on individual identification numbers contained in both data sources), or at a small-area level (for example, based on postal codes). In order to identify possible linkages, you may wish to expand the data source mapping exercise (STEP 2A) to include a list of possible data linkage criteria for each data source.

◉ **See**

"Harnessing small-area identifiers to link data for health inequality monitoring" on page 24

If data for health inequality monitoring can be obtained, proceed to STEP 3.

 If data for health inequality monitoring are not available, you may wish to begin the task of data collection; alternatively, you may reconsider your choices in STEP 1 (for example, selection of proxy indicators).

Examples and resources

 Data source mapping table templates

Template table 1. List data sources by type

Data source type	Data source name	Year(s) of data collection	Notes
Census			
Vital registration systems			
Household survey			
Administrative/facility data			
Surveillance systems			
Others [expand as required]			

Template table 2. List data sources and dimensions of inequality

No.	Data source and year [list all applicable]	Dimension of inequality [expand as required]			Notes
		[specify dimension]	[specify dimension]	[specify dimension]	
	Census (YEAR) [specify and expand list to include other years, as required]				
	Vital registration (YEAR) [specify years in operation]				
	Household survey (YEAR) [specify and expand list to include other years, as required]				
	Administrative/facility data (YEAR) [specify and expand list to include other years, as required]				
	Surveillance systems (YEAR) [specify and expand list to include other years, as required]				
	Other [specify and expand list to include other years, as required]				

Data source mapping table templates, continued

Template table 3. List health indicators and corresponding data sources

Health indicator [list all applicable]	Data source numbers [insert from table 2]	Notes
Indicator 1		
Indicator 2		
Indicator 3		
Indicator 4		
Indicator 5		
Indicator 6 [expand as required]		

Template table 4: Collate data from tables 2 and 3

Health indicator [list all applicable]	Dimension of inequality [expand as required] [insert corresponding data source numbers that appear in both tables 2 and 3]		
	[specify dimension]	[specify dimension]	[specify dimension]
Indicator 1			
Indicator 2			
Indicator 3			
Indicator 4			
Indicator 5			
Indicator 6 [expand as required]			

For more information about data source mapping and an example of its application to health inequality monitoring in the Philippines, see sections 2 and 5 of the World Health Organization *Handbook on health inequality monitoring: with a special focus on low- and middle-income countries*.

Major data sources and their strengths and limitations

Data for health inequality monitoring are commonly obtained from two major types of sources (population-based sources or institution-based sources) or, in the case of disease-specific registries, they may be obtained from surveillance systems. Common population-based data sources include censuses and vital registration systems (which are designed to cover all individuals in the population) and household surveys (which are typically designed to be representative of the population). Institution-based sources gather data in the course of administrative activities, covering only those members of the population who have interacted with the institution. An example of an institution-based data source is medical records. Surveillance systems usually provide detailed data on a single condition and/or from a single collection point.

When possible, collecting biometric data through blood testing or laboratory tests can be used to triangulate other forms of self-reported data or data related to diagnoses and treatment of diseases.

 For more information about major data sources used for health inequality monitoring, including the strengths and limitations of each, see section 2 of the World Health Organization *Handbook on health inequality monitoring: with a special focus on low- and middle-income countries*.

Harnessing small-area identifiers to link data for health inequality monitoring

Health inequality monitoring often draws from data collected at the individual level, however, in some settings where individual-level data are not available, data collected at the level of small-area geographical units may be a useful substitute. When health data contain a corresponding identifier, linkages may permit the merging of different data sources. For example, postal codes on individual medical records (which contain data about health indicators) can be linked with data about postal code-level socioeconomic status (data about dimensions of inequality such as median income, unemployment rate, median level of education, etc.). Deprivation indices have been developed that capture several types of socioeconomic characteristics (such as income, employment, housing, crime, education, access to services and living environment) by small-area geographical units (such as census tracts, electoral wards, postcode areas or municipalities). The Carstairs deprivation index, for example, is based on unemployment, overcrowding, car ownership and low social class.

- For more information about the use of area-based units for health inequality monitoring, see: Hosseinpoor AR, Bergen N. Area-based units of analysis for strengthening health inequality monitoring. Bull World Health. 2016;94(11):856–8.

STEP 3

Analyse data

STEP 3
Analyse data

A
Prepare disaggregated data

KEY QUESTION
What is the level of the health indicator in each population subgroup?

CHECKLIST
☐ Determine the level of the health indicator by subgroup (that is, disaggregated estimates)

B
Calculate summary measures of inequality

KEY QUESTION
What are the absolute and relative levels of health inequality?

CHECKLIST
☐ For each health indicator and dimension of inequality combination, calculate absolute inequality
☐ For each health indicator and dimension of inequality combination, calculate relative inequality

Overview

STEP ❸ of health inequality monitoring, data analysis, generates substantive content about health inequalities. The approach to data analysis described below begins with dividing the population into subgroups according to relevant dimensions of inequality and considering **disaggregated estimates** by these **population subgroups**. (Recall that populations are divided into subgroups based on the criteria identified in STEP 1C.) Disaggregated estimates show the situation in each population subgroup and can be used to assess patterns of inequality across socioeconomic subgroups.

Then, **summary measures of inequality** are calculated for each health indicator. Summary measures account for data from multiple subgroups to quantify health inequality in a single number, which can be used to make rapid comparisons of change in inequality over time, between indicators or across settings. Note that the components of STEPS 3A and 3B should be repeated for each dimension of inequality.

This step is the most technical, and we recommend that the step be informed by additional background reading about its theoretical basis and assumptions implicit in different types of summary measures. In addition, you may wish to explore publicly available statistical codes and tools that facilitate data analysis.

Section 3 of the World Health Organization *Handbook on health inequality monitoring: with a special focus on low- and middle-income countries* contains detailed explanations about the strengths and limitations of various summary measures.

A. Prepare disaggregated data

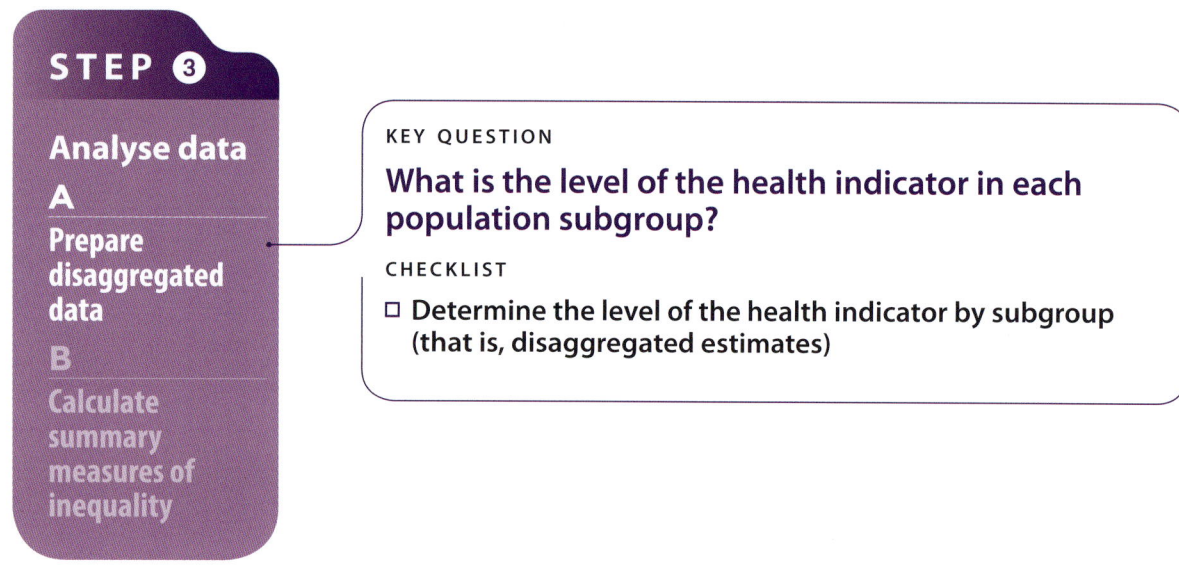

STEP 3

Analyse data

A Prepare disaggregated data

B Calculate summary measures of inequality

KEY QUESTION

What is the level of the health indicator in each population subgroup?

CHECKLIST

☐ **Determine the level of the health indicator by subgroup (that is, disaggregated estimates)**

Data analysis begins with the disaggregation of health data according to the dimensions of inequality. Each dimension of inequality will consist of at least two subgroups. Recall from STEP 1C that criteria specific to the dimensions of inequality should be applied to determine how they will be measured. Then, population subgroups can be formed. Dividing a population into subgroups may seem like a straightforward task; however, looking closely at how individuals are categorized reveals several nuanced issues. For example, subgroups based on economic status often divide the population into five quintiles, however, other options include using deciles or two groupings (such as poorest 40% vs remaining 60%). Place of residence is usually broken down as a binary of urban and rural areas, but other categorizations are also possible, such as main rural, remote rural, urban, semi-urban, etc. In forming subgroups by education, consider how many and which categories of education should be used. Similarly, how many and which categories of race or ethnicity should be applied? It may be useful to create a table to display the level of health by subgroup.

> **See**
>
> "Disaggregated data table template" on page 30

B. Calculate summary measures of inequality

STEP 3

Analyse data

A
Prepare disaggregated data

B
Calculate summary measures of inequality

KEY QUESTION

What are the absolute and relative levels of health inequality?

CHECKLIST

☐ For each health indicator and dimension of inequality combination, calculate absolute inequality

☐ For each health indicator and dimension of inequality combination, calculate relative inequality

The next stage of data analysis is the calculation of summary measures of inequality, drawing on disaggregated data from STEP 3A. There are two broad categories of summary measures: those that measure **absolute inequality** (reflecting the magnitude of inequality); and those that measure **relative inequality** (reflecting proportional inequality). When analysing data for health inequality monitoring, both absolute and relative summary measures should be used.

Within the two categories of absolute and relative measures, there are several different types of summary measures. The most straightforward measures – **simple measures of inequality** – draw on data from two subgroups, and include difference and ratio, which show absolute and relative inequality, respectively. **Complex measures of inequality** draw on data from more than two subgroups. Common complex measures that reflect absolute inequality include slope index of inequality, between group variance, mean difference from the mean and population attributable risk. Common complex measures that reflect relative inequality include concentration index, index of disparity, Theil index and population attributable fraction.

◎ **See**
"Statistical codes and tools that facilitate data analysis for health inequality monitoring" on page 30

◎ **See**
"Considerations for selecting appropriate summary measures of inequality" on page 31

Examples and resources

Disaggregated data table template

Dimensions of inequality	Health indicators		
	Indicator 1	Indicator 2	Indicator 3 *[expand as required]*
Dimension 1 Subgroup 1			
Dimension 1 Subgroup 2 *[expand as required]*			
Dimension 2 Subgroup 1			
Dimension 2 Subgroup 2 *[expand as required]*			
Dimension 3 Subgroup 1			
Dimension 3 Subgroup 2 *[expand as required]*			

Statistical codes and tools that facilitate data analysis for health inequality monitoring

The World Health Organization has coordinated the development of a number of statistical codes and tools that assist with data analysis for health inequality monitoring.

Statistical codes in R, Stata, SAS and SPSS allow for the calculation of disaggregated estimates from household survey data, taking into account survey sampling design.

- For more information about these statistical codes, see: http://www.who.int/gho/health_equity/statistical_codes/en/

The World Health Organization Health Equity Assessment Toolkit (HEAT) was developed to calculate summary measures of inequality using an existing database of disaggregated data. HEAT enables users to perform health inequality summary measure calculations using an existing database of disaggregated data, and to create customized visuals based on disaggregated data or summary measures. HEAT Plus, another edition of the HEAT software package, additionally allows users to upload and work with their own database.

- For more information about HEAT and HEAT Plus, see: http://www.who.int/gho/health_equity/assessment_toolkit/en/

Considerations for selecting appropriate summary measures of inequality

There are several types of considerations when deciding which summary measures of inequality are appropriate. Certain summary measures can show the level of inequality across **ordered subgroups** with a natural ranking (for example, economic status or education level), and other measures express inequality between subgroups that are **non-ordered** (for example, ethnicity or region). **Weighted summary measures** account for the subgroup population size, and **unweighted measure**s do not. Summary measures may require the use of a **reference group**, which provides a point of comparison when calculating health inequality. For example, measures of impact such as population attributable risk often define a reference group as the best performing or most advantaged subgroup.

 For more information about selecting appropriate summary measures of inequality, see section 3 of the World Health Organization *Handbook on health inequality monitoring: with a special focus on low- and middle-income countries*.

STEP 3

STEP 4

Report results

STEP 4
Report results

A
Define the target audience and purpose of reporting
KEY QUESTION
What parameters guide the approach to reporting?
CHECKLIST
- ☐ Define the overarching goals and objectives of reporting
- ☐ Identify the main audience for whom the report is prepared
- ☐ Determine the audience's prior knowledge of health inequalities and their level of technical expertise

B
Select the scope of reporting
KEY QUESTION
What aspects of the state of inequality should be covered by the report?
CHECKLIST
- ☐ Determine which data reflect the latest status of inequality
- ☐ Assess whether to report trend over time
- ☐ Assess whether to report benchmarking

C
Define the technical content of the report
KEY QUESTION
Which results of data analysis will be reported?
CHECKLIST
- ☐ Do an initial assessment of results to determine:
  - What are the most salient conclusions?
  - Are there any apparent patterns in the data?
- ☐ Report disaggregated data estimates
- ☐ Consider whether simple measures and complex measures reflect the same conclusions
  - If this is the case, it is generally recommended to report simple measures
  - If this is not the case, explore the reason for the discrepancy, and consider reporting complex measures, as appropriate, along with disaggregated estimates and other relevant information

D
Decide upon methods of presenting data
KEY QUESTION
How will key messages in the data be presented?
CHECKLIST
- ☐ Identify the appropriate tools to present the results:
  - text - tables - graphs - maps
- ☐ Consider using interactive visualization technology

E
Adhere to best practices of reporting
KEY QUESTION
What does the audience need to know to fully understand the context of the results?
CHECKLIST
- ☐ Report both absolute and relative inequality
- ☐ Indicate national average
- ☐ Indicate the population share of subgroups
- ☐ Flag results that are based on low sample size (if results are based on surveys)
- ☐ Consider reporting statistical significance, if appropriate
- ☐ Report the methods and process that underlie how you arrived at the conclusions

Overview

STEP ❹, building on the previous three steps, is to communicate the state of inequality to a specified audience. This reporting step brings together considerations about characteristics of the target audience and the purpose of reporting, as well as judgements about selecting and portraying the most salient results of the analysis step. Common outputs of reporting of health inequality monitoring include peer-reviewed articles (primarily targeted to academic and highly technical audiences), technical reports (targeted to technical audiences) and policy briefs (targeted to policy-makers).

In this step, consider the anticipated impact that you hope to achieve through reporting, keeping in mind the ultimate goal of health inequality monitoring: to help to inform policies, programmes and practices to reduce inequality. A thorough assessment and understanding of the results of the analyses will help to ensure that reporting choices capture an appropriate depiction of the state of inequality, and account for the inherent limitations of summary measures.

For more information about the fourth step of health inequality monitoring, see section 4 of the World Health Organization *Handbook on health inequality monitoring: with a special focus on low- and middle-income countries*.

A. Define the target audience and purpose of reporting

STEP 4

Report results

A
Define the target audience and purpose of reporting

B
Select the scope of reporting

C
Define the technical content of the report

D
Decide upon methods of presenting data

E
Adhere to best practices of reporting

KEY QUESTION
What parameters guide the approach to reporting?

CHECKLIST
☐ Define the overarching goals and objectives of reporting
☐ Identify the main audience for whom the report is prepared
☐ Determine the audience's prior knowledge of health inequalities and their level of technical expertise

When reporting health inequality data, begin by defining the overarching goals and objectives for the report. This helps to ensure that all subsequent reporting decisions remain in line with these aims, and that the final report is prepared in a way that focuses on achieving the stated purpose.

Reporting may entail communicating information to government officials, researchers, public health practitioners, policy-makers and/or others. The target audience should always be considered when deciding how to report data, as different audiences have different levels of understanding, technical expertise and requirements of what they need to take away from the report. Having a clear understanding of the audience, including their abilities and needs, will help to make the communication of results more effective, and inform subsequent decisions that follow the reporting step.

B. Select the scope of reporting

STEP 4

Report results

A
Define the target audience and purpose of reporting

**B
Select the scope of reporting**

C
Define the technical content of the report

D
Decide upon methods of presenting data

E
Adhere to best practices of reporting

KEY QUESTION
What aspects of the state of inequality should be covered by the report?

CHECKLIST
☐ Determine which data reflect the latest status of inequality
☐ Assess whether to report trend over time
☐ Assess whether to report benchmarking

The next stage involves selecting the scope of reporting. At a minimum, reports about the state of inequality should present the latest status of inequality. The latest status of inequality is derived from the latest available data, and addresses questions such as: What is the situation? How is the country (or other geographical area of interest) doing? And what should be current priorities for action? If data availability allows and it falls within the defined objectives, then reporting may also encompass trends in inequality over time and benchmarking.

Reporting time trends helps to identify whether inequality has improved or worsened over time. While time trends do not directly address the question of whether a policy or programme has made an impact – more complex and detailed studies would be necessary for this – they can be valuable for policy-makers to gauge whether change is warranted. Health inequality monitoring can and should be closely linked to policy and programme evaluation.

Benchmarking is the process of comparing data from similar countries to get an idea of one country's level of inequality in relation to others, and helps to give additional context to the state of inequality. Depending upon the scope of the monitoring activity and health topic, benchmarking can also be conducted on a smaller scale. For example, the province level of wealth-related health inequality can be compared across provinces.

C. Define the technical content of the report

STEP 4

Report results

A
Define the target audience and purpose of reporting

B
Select the scope of reporting

C
Define the technical content of the report

D
Decide upon methods of presenting data

E
Adhere to best practices of reporting

KEY QUESTION

Which results of data analysis will be reported?

CHECKLIST

- **Do an initial assessment of results to determine:**
  - What are the most salient conclusions?
  - Are there any apparent patterns in the data?
- **Report disaggregated data estimates**
- **Consider whether simple measures and complex measures reflect the same conclusions**
  - If this is the case, it is generally recommended to report simple measures
  - If this is not the case, explore the reason for the discrepancy, and consider reporting complex measures, as appropriate, along with disaggregated estimates and other relevant information

> **See**
> "A systematic approach to defining priority areas based on the results of health inequality monitoring" on page 41

> **See**
> "Characteristic patterns of inequality across disaggregated data" on page 41

The technical content contained in the report should support the major themes and conclusions. It should also cater to the audience, purpose and scope of the report. Determining appropriate technical content for a report requires a thorough understanding of the limitations of summary measures of inequality, and a careful assessment of the results.

In general, it is recommended to report the most straightforward technical content wherever possible. Including disaggregated estimates in reports is often an appropriate way to highlight patterns of inequality, especially if inequality presents as a gradient across socioeconomic subgroups. Disaggregated data should be reported to support the conclusions presented in a report. In addition, consider whether simple measures of inequality reflect the same conclusions as complex measures. For instance, a simple measure of inequality is preferable over a complex measure, provided that they support the same conclusion. If this is not the case, then a complex measure may be warranted to provide more context about the situation, if appropriate for the audience and report purpose. Identify any discrepancies, and determine how to put the results in context, including their application in policy and programmatic settings. When relevant, it may be warranted to report information in addition to disaggregated data and summary measures, such as the share of the affected population in each subgroup or how the **population share** has shifted over time.

D. Decide upon methods of presenting data

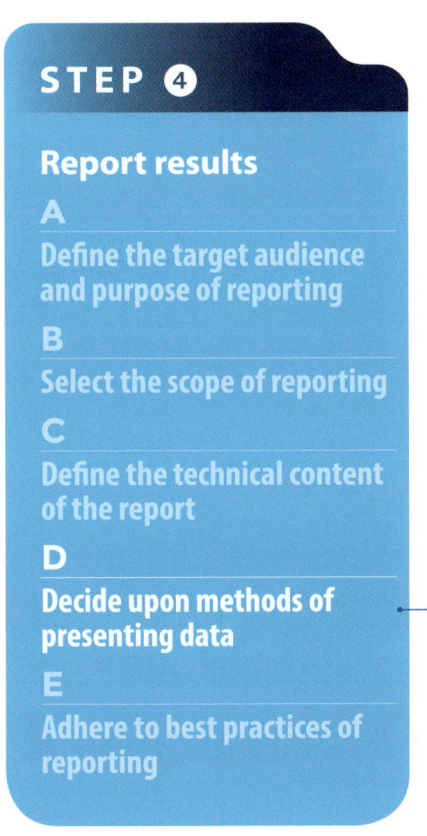

STEP 4

Report results

A Define the target audience and purpose of reporting

B Select the scope of reporting

C Define the technical content of the report

D Decide upon methods of presenting data

E Adhere to best practices of reporting

KEY QUESTION
How will key messages in the data be presented?

CHECKLIST
- **Identify the appropriate tools to present the results:**
  - text
  - tables
  - graphs
  - maps
- **Consider using interactive visualization technology**

Data presentation should be deliberate and comprehensible, and convey the appropriate amount and scope of data to the target audience. The nature of the data and the needs of the audience should drive the choice of the visualization technique. Less technically minded audiences may benefit from simpler graphs and summarizing texts, whereas more technically minded audiences may wish to engage with more comprehensive presentations of data. For instance, text can be effective in explaining nuances and patterns in the data, and often serves to complement other types of data presentation tools. Tables state data values explicitly, and provide a precise and comprehensive overview of data; however, they tend to require a large effort from the reader to derive conclusions. Graphs can be effective in simplifying complex messages, and conveying large amounts of data at once. Using a variety of graphs to introduce data can help to display the message in different ways; however, it is generally best to stick to one or two types of graphs to maintain consistency throughout the report. Maps can be appropriate to show data with a geographical component, though keep in mind that the size of the country or region may not correspond with the population size or density.

The use of data visualization technology opens possibilities for new and evolving ways of reporting data, including interactive options. Data visualization can be created using a range of software, from widely available software with many applications, to more specialized statistical software and visual analytics software. For instance, HEAT and HEAT Plus allow users to generate customized visual outputs.

See
"Statistical codes and tools that facilitate data analysis for health inequality monitoring" on page 30

E. Adhere to best practices of reporting

STEP 4

Report results

A. Define the target audience and purpose of reporting

B. Select the scope of reporting

C. Define the technical content of the report

D. Decide upon methods of presenting data

E. Adhere to best practices of reporting

KEY QUESTION

What does the audience need to know to fully understand the context of the results?

CHECKLIST

- ☐ Report both absolute and relative inequality
- ☐ Indicate national average
- ☐ Indicate the population share of subgroups
- ☐ Flag results that are based on low sample size (if results are based on surveys)
- ☐ Consider reporting statistical significance, if appropriate
- ☐ Report the methods and process that underlie how you arrived at the conclusions

The final component of reporting is a quality check, to ensure that the best practices of reporting have been fulfilled. All of the practices listed above communicate information that helps to put the results in context. These practices also make the reporting process more transparent and thorough, which provides a stronger case to urge remedial action where needed. For instance, reporting the size of the subgroups, where warranted, can highlight where results are based on low sample sizes (which may not accurately capture the situation and/or may be meaningless). Reporting the confidence interval of point estimates can be useful to help audiences understand whether health indicators are statistically different between subgroups. The interpretation of confidence intervals, however, should be done carefully when estimates are derived from large sample sizes. Estimates based on large sample sizes are more likely to be statistically different mathematically; however, in some cases, the difference may have little implication for public health. For instance, a 2 percentage point difference in coverage of a health intervention between rural and urban areas (such as 80% vs 82%) may prove to be statistically significant, however, this difference may be of little practical importance to public health.

Examples and resources

A systematic approach to defining priority areas based on the results of health inequality monitoring

A straightforward and intuitive interpretation of health inequality monitoring helps policy-makers and other stakeholders (including the public) to understand the results of inequality analyses in light of planned national targets, health-care agendas and other contextual factors. A systematic approach to consolidate the results of inequality monitoring may be a useful starting point when defining priority areas. One approach, detailed in section 4.7 of the *Handbook on health inequality monitoring: with a special focus on low- and middle-income countries*, involves a three-point scoring system of the results. Briefly, the approach accounts for the large amounts of data across all health indicators by each dimension of inequality, assigning a score at each intersecting point and for national averages. Scores are determined through agreement of those involved in the health inequality monitoring process. Tallying the scores for each health indicator and dimension of inequality provides a numerical output that may help to illustrate possible policy priorities. We note that this somewhat prescriptive process is not intended to generate an indisputable ranking of priority areas; rather, it is intended to serve as one form of evidence for the complex process of creating policy.

 For more information about defining priority areas and an example of its application to health inequality monitoring in the Philippines, see sections 4 and 5 of the World Health Organization *Handbook on health inequality monitoring: with a special focus on low- and middle-income countries*.

Characteristic patterns of inequality across disaggregated data

For dimensions of inequality that can be ranked, disaggregated data across subgroups may demonstrate characteristic patterns of inequality. Examining inequality across subgroups is an important aspect of national monitoring, revealing patterns in disaggregated data and generating evidence to support appropriate policy and targeting.

Four characteristic patterns of inequality have been identified. A pattern of mass deprivation occurs where a large proportion of the population performs poorly (such as low coverage of a health intervention) and only a small proportion performs well. A pattern of mass deprivation may indicate a need for policies with a broad, population-wide focus. A pattern of marginal exclusion is evident where only a small proportion of the population performs poorly, and most of the population performs well. This scenario can be best addressed through a targeted focus on the most disadvantaged subgroup. Queuing patterns show an incremental increase across subgroups. This scenario requires a combination of focusing on the population-at-large, with special targeting of the most disadvantaged. A pattern of complete coverage is observed when all subgroups perform well. Here, ongoing monitoring is warranted to ensure that the situation is maintained.

- For more information and examples, see: Hosseinpoor AR, Bergen N, Koller T, Prasad A, Schlotheuber A, Valentine N et al. Equity-oriented monitoring in the context of universal health coverage. PLoS Med. 2014;11(9):e1001727.

Glossary

Absolute inequality reflects the magnitude of difference in health between subgroups. Absolute measures of inequality retain the same unit of measure as the health indicator.

Benchmarking is the process of comparing data from similar areas or populations to get an idea of how one area/population performs in relation to others. Benchmarking provides context for a broader understanding of the state of inequality.

Complex measures of inequality draw on data from all subgroups to produce a single number that is an expression of the level of inequality. For example, they can express inequality across all wealth quintiles, or among all regions in a country.

A **composite indicator** is an index composed of several indicators within a health topic to represent that topic; a composite indicator may also combine indicators from several different health topics (for example, forming an index to measure universal health coverage).

Data source mapping is a systematic process for cataloguing and describing all data that are available for health inequality monitoring in a given context. The process can be broken down into four sequential stages: (1) list available data sources by type; (2) for each data source, determine availability of data for dimensions of inequality; (3) for each data source, determine availability of data about health indicators; and (4) combine the lists about health indicators and dimensions of inequality. Note that this is a recommended approach, and that any of the stages may be modified to suit the needs of the user.

A **dimension of inequality** is the categorization upon which subgroups are formed for health inequality monitoring, such as wealth, education, region, sex, etc. The selection of dimensions of inequality typically includes categories that are reasonably likely to reflect unfair differences between groups that could be corrected by changes to policies, programmes or practices.

Disaggregated estimates are data that are broken down by population subgroups (as opposed to overall average).

Double disaggregation is the practice of filtering data according to two dimensions of inequality simultaneously. Double disaggregation permits exploration of intersectionality.

Equity stratifier – *see: dimension of inequality*.

Health inequalities are observable health differences between subgroups within a population. Health inequalities can be measured and monitored.

Health inequity is a normative concept that describes systematic differences in health between population subgroups that are deemed to be unjust, unfair and avoidable. Health inequity is linked to forms of disadvantage that are socially produced, such as poverty, discrimination and lack of access to services or goods.

Linked data, in the context of health inequality monitoring, are data about health indicators and dimensions of inequality that stem from different data sources, and are merged through an individual or small-area characteristic.

Monitoring is a process of repeatedly observing a situation to watch for changes over time. While monitoring can help to determine the impact of policies, programmes and practices, monitoring alone cannot typically explain the cause of troublesome trends. Rather, monitoring may be thought of as a warning system. Monitoring activities can both inform and direct research in a given area. Because monitoring tracks progress over time, it can be described as a continual cycle.

The **Monitoring, Evaluation and Review Framework**, developed by the World Health Organization, organizes health indicators into four components: inputs and processes; outputs; outcomes; and impact. Within each component, various categories of indicators are defined that allow the measurement of health at many levels. Indicators of inputs and processes are broad, affecting many other parts of the health sector. Indicators that fall under outputs and outcomes tend to be quite specific to a particular health topic, and may respond quickly to changes and progress in the health sector. Impact indicators, which are slower to respond to policy, programme and practice changes, are important to provide a snapshot of the health of a population.

Non-ordered inequality dimensions are not based on criteria that can be logically ranked. For example, region, ethnicity and religion dimensions of inequality typically contain subgroups that are non-ordered.

Ordered inequality dimensions have an inherent positioning and can be logically ranked. For example, wealth and education level are dimensions of inequality that typically contain subgroups that can be ordered.

Population share describes the percentage of the population that is represented by a given population subgroup. In cases where the health indicator does not affect the entire population, population share expresses the percentage of the *affected* population represented by a given population subgroup. For example, if looking at service coverage among pregnant women, then population share would express the percentage of pregnant women in a given subgroup out of all pregnant women in the population.

Population subgroups, in the context of health inequality monitoring, reflect ways of grouping a population based on a dimension of inequality. For example, population subgroups based on wealth are commonly grouped as quintiles, ranging from the poorest 20% to the richest 20%.

Proxy indicators stand in for other indicators that are difficult to measure, or for which data are limited.

A **reference group** provides a point of comparison when calculating health inequality, and is a feature of certain types of summary measures of inequality. For example, measures of impact such as population attributable risk often define a reference group as the best performing or most advantaged subgroup.

Relative inequality shows the proportional differences in health among subgroups. Relative measures of inequality are unit-less.

Simple measures of inequality make pairwise comparisons of health between two subgroups, such as the most and least wealthy. These are the most commonly used measures in inequality monitoring, as they are intuitive and easily understood. Simple measures of inequality are typically unweighted.

Summary measures of inequality yield a single number that reflects the level of inequality between two or more subgroups. Summary measures of inequality may indicate absolute or relative inequality, and may involve two subgroups (that is, simple pairwise measures) or more than two subgroups (that is, complex measures). Summary measures of inequality may be weighted or unweighted.

A **tracer indicator** is a specified health indicator chosen to represent a broader health topic. Tracer indicators have the advantage of being easy to understand and report, but may lead to more resources being dedicated to an area simply because it is being monitored.

Unweighted measures treat each subgroup as equally sized, and is a feature of simple measures of inequality and certain complex measures of inequality.

Weighted measures take into account the population size of each subgroup. This is a feature of certain complex measures of inequality.